Low Fat Diet

Low Fat Cooking with Gluten Free and Paleo Recipes

Judy Keating

Copyright © 2013 Judy Keating
All rights reserved.

Table of Contents

LOW FAT DIET INTRODUCTION 1

SECTION 1: GLUTEN FREE VEGAN 6

WHAT IS GLUTEN? 8
    Celiac Disease 8

VEGAN LIFESTYLE AND DIET 11
    History..11
    Philosophy...11

GLUTEN FREE VEGAN ALTERNATIVE INGREDIENTS . 13
    Eggs..13
    Flour...14
    Butter..16
    Milk Substitutes 17
    Vegan Pasta..18
    Gluten Free Vegan Pie Crust...19

GLUTEN FREE VEGAN RECIPES................................... 21

SNACKS 21
    Onion Rings 21
    Sweet Potato Fries..23
    Peanut Butter Apple (quick snack)..24

MAIN DISHES 25
    Vegetables and Rice...25
    Chickpea Salad..27
    Pasta Marinara...28
    Simple Mexican Stew 30
    Simple Spanish Rice 31

Vegetable Pot Pie 33

SIDE DISHES 35
Potato Rice Balls 35
Vegan Baked Potato 36
Chestnut Rissoles 38
Polenta and Corn 39

DESSERTS 41
Zucchini Banana Spice Cake 41
Creamy Apple Tapioca 43
Strawberries in Cherry Syrup 44
Banana Nut Bread 45
Vegan Gluten Free Chocolate Chip Cookies 47

SOUPS 49
Gluten Free Vegan Tomato Soup 49
Hearty Mexican Soup 51
Potato, Squash and Apple Soup 52
French Cabbage Soup 53

RAW FOODS, SEASONAL FAVORITES AND DRINKS ... 54
Pineapple Banana Drink 54
Bacon- Sort Of! 55
"Eggnog" 56
Vegan Cocoa 57
Holiday Favorite Pumpkin Pie 58

GLUTEN FREE VEGAN STAPLES FOR THE PANTRY ... 59

HEALTH CONCERNS OF A VEGAN GLUTEN FREE DIET 61
Vitamin B-12 61
Iron 62
Omega-3 Fatty Acids 63
Calcium 63
Gluten Free Concerns 64

GLUTEN FREE VEGAN CONCLUSION 66

VEGAN FAQ'S 67
Is a vegan diet healthy? 67
How difficult is it to go vegan? 67
Is a vegan diet expensive? 67

GLUTEN FREE FAQ'S 69
What foods can I eat? 69
Why are oats such a big deal? 69
Is celiac disease really that bad? 69

GLUTEN FREE VEGAN -- IN SUMMARY 72

SECTION 2: PALEOLITHIC COOKBOOK 74

WHAT IS PALEO? 76

WHY GO THE PALEOLITHIC DIET ROUTE? 78

BENEFITS OF THE PALEO LIFESTYLE 79

PALEO FOOD TYPES 81
Foods to eat 81
Foods to avoid 82

PALEO CONFUSION 83
How to know if a food type adheres to the paleo plan. 83

PALEO FOOD LIST 84

SAMPLE DAILY MEAL PLAN FOR BEGINNERS 88

v

EATING PALEO IN DAY TO DAY LIFE ... 89
- Restaurants and Eating Out ... 89
- Social Eating ... 90
- Food Preparation ... 91
- Meal Frequency and Amounts ... 91

RECIPE IDEAS ... 93

BREAKFAST ... 93
- Mushroom and Pine Nuts Scrambled Eggs ... 93
- Salmon and Zucchini Fritters ... 94
- Lemon Pancakes ... 96

LUNCH RECIPES ... 97
- Dory Fillet with Beetroot Salad ... 97
- Cucumber Hot Dogs ... 98

DINNER RECIPES ... 100
- Chicken Curry with Pumpkin ... 100

SIDES ... 102

SOUPS AND SALADS ... 102
- Broccoli and Pine Nut Soup ... 102
- Roast Vegetables in Orange and Rosemary ... 104

MEATS ... 105
- Crunchy Sweet Potato Chips with Meatballs ... 105
- Peppered Steak ... 107
- Paprika Lamb ... 108
- Moroccan Lamb with Squash ... 110

POULTRY ... 112
- Chicken with Macadamia Topping ... 112
- Orange Chicken with Basil ... 114
- Avocado Sauce with Baked Chicken ... 115

Bombay Chicken Skewers 117

SNACKS 120
Pistachio Salsa..120
Tomato Salsa..121
Cashew Nut Dip 122
Desserts 123
Mixed Berry Compote..124

PALEOLITHIC COOKBOOK CONCLUSION 126

Low Fat Diet Introduction

A low fat diet is a nutritious diet that does more than just help a person to lose unwanted fat and weight. There is a difference in fats, so let's be clear here that we are talking about "bad" fats, fats that stick to the body and cause weight to pile on. Good fats like fatty acids and those found in oils like olive oil are very beneficial to the body. This book is not about reducing the intake of "good" fats, but of lowering the bad unhealthy fats. An effective weight loss plan will include a good balance of all the nutrients, including healthy fats.

If a person wants to go on a low fat diet, they may opt to buy prepackaged foods labeled as "low fat" or "reduced fat." What many of these products fail to say is that they remove the good fat in order to label it as such, so you really have to watch what you purchase and eat if you go that route. Many "low fat" prepackaged foods are full of sugar, which for all intents and purposes, is a low fat food, just that it is not a good food. Sugar does turn to fat in the body, so while it may not contain fat, it will eventually become fat, on your thighs, belly, upper arms. A true low fat diet will be one with reduced calories. Do not fall for low fat labels. You are better off making your meals from scratch, that way you can see each ingredient you add and know that it is fresh and whole.

Keep in mind that you need healthy fats in your diet, these are the unsaturated fats found naturally in foods like salmon and other fish, and in certain oils like canola and olive. These fats work with the body to facilitate weight loss and in helping to boost brain function and strengthen the immune system. They give energy, which encourages movement, and movement is good for weight loss. The more energy you have the more you will move and exercise. Do not reduce the intake of foods with healthy fats; instead think in terms to reduce the size of the portions of foods that may contain "bad" fats.

Sometimes it is very difficult to cut out all fat from the diet. When you know the food has a good amount of fat just greatly reduce the size of the portion you eat. Eat more of the food you know is healthier. Opt for a smaller cut of meat and choose another spoon of steamed vegetables or another piece of fruit.

If you eat a low fat diet the right way, you will lose

weight at a nice steady pace. If you make low fat dieting a means to lose weight you also need to make a lifestyle change to keep the weight off. If you diet just long enough to lose the weight then go back to eating the same way you did before the weight will pile right back on the body. Once you lose the weight on a low fat diet, you need to modify the diet to maintain the weight loss. Do not stay on a very low fat diet indefinitely. Instead try to follow the diet plans in this book, modify it to include a few more calories and the weight will stay off, especially if you couple it with exercise.

Each of the diets featured in this book offers low fat recipes to help facilitate weight loss. Each diet goes with two very distinctive and different lifestyles, one being a strict vegetarian, or vegan and the other includes many meat choices. Whichever camp you are in you can find enough recipes in this book to plan meals for several weeks.

A sampling of the recipes from the Gluten Free Vegan Diet include: From the Snacks section try the Sweet Potato Fries, Onion Rings and Peanut Butter Apple. From the side dishes, try Potato Rice Balls, Chestnut Rissoles, Vegan Baked Potato and Polenta and Corn. From the main dishes, try Simple Spanish Rice, Vegetable Pot Pie, Pasta Marinara, Chickpea Salad and Simple Mexican

Stew. From the desserts section try Creamy Apple Tapioca, Banana Nut Bread, Strawberries in Cherry Syrup and Vegan Gluten Free Chocolate Chip Cookies. From the soups section try the Hearty Mexican Soup, French Cabbage Soup, Potato, Squash and Apple Soup and the Gluten Free Vegan Tomato Soup. From the "Raw Foods, Seasonal Favorites and Drinks" section try the Eggnog (eggless of course!), Vegan Cocoa, Pineapple Banana Drink and the Holiday Favorite Pumpkin Pie. You can see you have a great deal to choose from including the delicious sweetness of desserts.

The Paleo Diet has many good recipes, which are heavy on the meat side, so this is a good diet for meat lovers. Try the Mushroom and Pine Nuts Scrambled Eggs or the Salmon and Zucchini Fritters from the breakfast section. For meat lovers here are a sampling of some of the savory and delicious meat recipes: Peppered Steak, Bombay Chicken Skewers, Crunchy Sweet Potato Chips with Meatball, Moroccan Lamb with Squash, Chicken with Macadamia Topping, and Avocado Sauce with Baked Chicken and a delicious Orange Chicken with Basil. Even the Paleo diet has a delicious snacks and dessert section, try the Cashew Nut Dip or the Mixed Berry Compote.

Always seek the advice and counsel of your health care

provider before starting any new diet plan. Go over any medications you are taking and ask about adding exercise, especially if you are doing this to lose weight. Weight loss happens faster if you couple a low fat diet with exercise. Being physical at least every other day for half an hour a day is very vital to your well-being. Both diet and exercise should be continued once the desired weight is gone, however adjust the low fat to include a few more "healthy" carbs.

Section 1: Gluten Free Vegan

It seems as if every time you turn around there is another diet plan being touted as the miracle answer to all that ails you, especially excessive weight. Gluten free and vegan diets do not necessarily fall into this category! Each has become progressively more popular, however the reasons behind this type of lifestyle change goes far beyond losing weight.

There are many different reasons people consider drastic changes to their diet and lifestyle. Many times health is a major motivator, especially when it comes to eliminating gluten from your daily diet. Here are a few common reasons individuals choose to live a gluten free vegan lifestyle:

- You are a vegan and discovered you have gluten intolerance or celiac disease
- You are concerned with the ethical treatment of animals slaughtered for meat production
- You want a healthier diet filled with rich, live foods (plants do not have to die to provide a meal.)
- Meat and processed foods are expensive

- You have suffered various ailments over the years that are only alleviated with a gluten free diet

If you have been considering this shift in eating habits, you should understand what it means to be vegan and how gluten can cause various issues for someone who is sensitive to wheat proteins.

What is Gluten?

Gluten is a protein found in foods processed from wheat and related grains. Many people are shocked to learn just how many items at the grocery store contain gluten or are gluten contaminated. For many people this is not a big deal, but for those who suffer from gluten sensitivity or celiac disease, it is a very big deal indeed.

Celiac Disease

In many circles the use of the phrases gluten intolerance and celiac disease are used interchangeably, however recent research suggests intolerance may have a much broader scope than celiac disease. To date, however, many medical journals may use the terms interchangeably.

What is gluten intolerance or celiac disease? If you are sensitive to gluten the sensitive villi in your digestive tract can become damaged when you consume gluten laden products via an allergic type reaction in which the immune system attacks the lining of your digestive tract. The exact cause of the disease is unknown and can develop at any age.

Symptoms:

- Abdominal pain- bloating, gas or heartburn
- Nausea and vomiting
- Changes in appetite (up or down)
- Foul stool that floats, appears fatty or shows evidence of blood
- Depression
- Hair loss
- Skin rashes
- Joint pain and aches
- Brain fog
- Chronic constipation
- Fatigue
- Changes to menstrual cycle
- Stunted growth
- Tingling or numbness in hands and feet

It is important to note that these are but a few symptoms, not a comprehensive list. Furthermore you may suffer few, many or be completely asymptomatic.

If all of this is sounding familiar, you may want to begin the diagnostic process with a self test, which is really just asking yourself some basic questions related to major symptoms. If you are dealing with four or more symptoms, it is time to talk to your physician as you may have a gluten sensitivity issue. Your doctor will want to run a series of tests to confirm your diagnosis, before you change your eating habits.

Vegan Lifestyle and Diet

Vegan and vegetarian are quite similar, but with a few pronounced differences. Some would say that a vegan diet is merely a stricter form of vegetarianism, and to some extent that is true. However, practitioners feel a vegan lifestyle is as much a philosophy as it is a diet plan.

History

Vegetarianism has been around since at least the 19th century, and the first vegan cookbook was published in 1910. Nevertheless, the word vegan was not coined until 1944 when a couple members of the Leicester Vegetarian Society expressed concern over the fact that vegetarians were still consuming dairy products. The first vegan society in the United States was founded in 1948.

Philosophy

Veganism has a "mission" (for lack of a better phrase) statement that sum up this particular groups beliefs and motivations.

"The doctrine that man should live without exploiting animals." This means that in addition to meat being stricken from the menu, for example:

- Meat- (goes without saying)
- Eggs- it is a baby chicken after all
- Honey- bees are taken advantage of for human consumption.

Concern for the ethical treatment of farm animals is but one reason people turn to a vegan lifestyle. Recent studies suggest a cause and effect relationship between the consumption of red meat and increased incidences of colon cancer. Add to that the concerns about growth hormones in chicken and the use of a multitude of drugs in cattle, pork and chickens, it is not really difficult to see why more and more people are second guessing their diets and lifestyles.

Of course, opting for a vegan diet, particularly one that is gluten free is not exactly easy! However, with the right recipes and a little encouragement you will soon find yourself on the way to a healthier and more environmentally friendly life.

Gluten Free Vegan Alternative Ingredients

One of the biggest challenges with a gluten free vegan diet is finding recipes that are tasty and satisfying. The list of prohibited foods is long, but you can still create delicious meals and even some family favorites by substituting ingredients and learning to use fragrant spices and colorful vegetables in your dishes. Let's start by discussing some vegan and gluten free substitutes for popular ingredients.

Eggs

Eggs are a great source of protein and a common binding agent in a myriad of recipes. Thankfully, you can use several replacement ingredients, depending on the type of dish you are creating. A few examples include:

Sweet Dishes- Cakes, cookies and other desserts

- Applesauce- ¼ cup for each egg
- Vinegar and Baking powder- when you have a

recipe calling for three or more eggs, you can use this substitute: 1 tablespoon each vinegar, water and baking powder.
- Potato Starch- 2 heaping tablespoons
- Pureed banana- ¼ cup per egg (for lighter cakes the conversion is 3 tablespoons per egg)
- Water- ¼ cup per egg
- Soy Yogurt- ¼ per egg
- Arrowroot- 2 heaping teaspoons per egg
- Binding Agents- non-desert recipes
- 2-3 Tablespoons- mashed potato flakes, arrowroot powder or tomato paste
- Vegetable Oil- ¼ cup per egg
- Flax Seed- 1 tablespoon ground seed to 3 tablespoons of water (great source of omega 3's)

Flour

If you like to bake cakes, cookies and breads you will need gluten free flour substitutes. You might be inclined to think you can just grab a gluten free alternative off the shelf and substitute it cup for cup in your favorite recipe, however it is not quite that simple. Gluten free alternatives have different textures, flavors and fat contents. For example coconut flour absorbs water like crazy and almond flour has a distinct flavor.

A good alternative is to create your own all-purpose flour mixture.

Alternative Flour Mixture:

1 ½ cup millet flour
1 ½ cup sorghum flour
1 ¾ cup potato starch

As you begin creating your own dishes you will probably want to tinker with the above mixture, feel free to mix and match ingredients and amounts until you find the perfect all-purpose flour alternative for your favorite dishes.

Gluten Free Flours

Bean Flours:

- Kinako- roasted soy flour
- Garbanzo bean
- Fava bean
- White Flours
- Sweet rice
- White rice
- Tapioca

- Nut Flours
- Coconut
- Almond
- Chestnut
- Whole Grain
- Brown rice
- Quinoa
- Teff

In the beginning your recipes will be more like mini-adventures, but that is half the fun! Why make gluten free vegan living a boring endeavor? If you happen to opt for dark buckwheat as a gluten free flour alternative, you should know your dish will have a decided purple hue.

Butter

Butter has several roles in baking, it can act as a binding agent, leavening agent, adds flavor and sometimes texture. However, since it is a dairy product it must be stricken from the vegan shopping list. Thankfully it is fairly easy to replace. Here are a few options:

Butter to Olive Oil:

1 teaspoon- ¾ teaspoon
1 tablespoon- 2 ¼ teaspoon
¼ cup- 3 tablespoons

For cookies or recipes where creamed butter is required coconut oil is a better option. You can use identical quantities and then simply beat the coconut butter to a semi-solid state. Other butter substitutes include but are not limited to:

Untoasted sesame seed oil
Vegan shortening
Canola oil

Milk Substitutes

Probably one of the easiest substitutions to make today as there are already a number of non-dairy alternatives available at your local grocery store. A few you might want to consider include:

Almond Milk
Soy Milk
Coconut milk
Non-dairy powdered milk
Meat Substitutes

Not all vegans are interested in substituting for meat, however if you would still like the occasional burger or do not fancy spaghetti with sauce alone, you may want some alternatives. One thing you have to watch with popular commercial vegan meat substitutes is the wheat content. For the gluten free vegan diet, you will have to stick with soy and tofu based alternatives, but make sure you read the ingredients list. Tofu is generally the go to meat replacement as it is basically tasteless and will take on the flavor of whatever seasonings you use in your dish.

Now that you have some idea of what you should add to your shopping list, it is time to get on with some tasty recipes! Here are a few tried and tested gluten free vegan recipes you can add to your recipe caddy.

Vegan Pasta

2 cups chickpea flour
12 tablespoons water
4 tablespoons ground flaxseed

Mix together flaxseed and warm water, gently whisk ingredients together and set aside. On your cutting /

rolling board, pour your chickpea flour, making a mound of sorts. Create a well in the center. Once the flaxseed mixture has jelled, (five minutes or so) pour in the middle of your flour well.

Mix chickpea flour and flaxseed together gently, forming a dough ball. Wrap in plastic wrap and allow to sit at room temperature for approximately half an hour.

The key to making tasty pasta with chickpea flour is getting the dough rolled thin enough, which can be a challenge. If you plan to do this the old fashioned way, (roller and countertop) make sure to use small portions of the dough at a time. Roll very thin, cut into squares and create bowtie pasta. (Easiest pasta form to make without a pasta machine)

Gluten Free Vegan Pie Crust

1 ½ cup rice flour or other gluten free alternative (some flours will be sweeter than others)
½-cup shortening- (may substitute vegan margarine)
4 tablespoons water

Create dough balls by cutting shortening or alternative into the flour until you have a crumbly mixture. Gently form into balls and then either roll flat with your rolling pin or form it to your pie pan by hand. Bake in oven for 10-15 minutes at 400 degrees.

Gluten Free Vegan Recipes

Snacks

No matter how healthy your diet may be, snacks are probably a part of your daily routine. If not, once you get a load of these tasty, yet gluten free vegan alternatives, you will change your mind.

Onion Rings

If onion rings are your sole purpose for hitting the fast food drive through, you are in luck with this first snack. Not only is it easy to prepare and cost effective, it tastes great and you can enjoy it any time day or night from the comfort of your own home.

1 med onion- sweet Vidalia's are a good option
¼ cup soy milk (almond works as well)
½ cup coconut flour
Season to Taste- cayenne pepper, salt, garlic seasoning, onion powder etc…

Slice your onion carefully, laying aside intact rings. Place milk and flour in separate bowls, adding your preferred seasonings to the flour. Dip each ring first in milk and then in the flour, being careful to fully coat each ring. Lay rings separately on a non-stick baking pan. Bake for 20 minutes at 450°.

Sweet Potato Fries

McDonald's may have some of the best French fries on the market today, but they cannot hold a candle to sweet potato fries! Healthy and great tasting, why opt for a greasy high calorie alternative?

1-3 medium sweet potatoes
1-2 teaspoons coconut oil
1 tablespoon equal parts cinnamon/ sugar (check labels for gluten free processed spices)

Peel and slice sweet potatoes, making strips of raw potatoes (fries). Place fries in a single layer on a non-stick baking sheet. Drizzle fries with coconut oil and sprinkle lavishly with sugar/ cinnamon mixture. Bake fries for approximately 30 minutes at 425°. For added snacking pleasure dust warm fries with powdered sugar.

Peanut Butter Apple (quick snack)

Sometimes you want a tasty snack but do not have the time to slice, cook and wait! For those occasions sliced apples and a peanut butter dip can really hit the spot.

½ cup peanut butter
Dash of coconut milk
Pinch of cinnamon

First, choose your apples, Fuji and gala are probably the most common peel and eat apples, but if you like, something with a bit more bite a granny smith will work.

In a medium mixing bowl combine ingredients and beat on medium speed until your peanut butter dip is nice and creamy. Peel, core and slice your apples. Voila, you have a tasty snack you can whip up in a hurry.

TIP: If you are in a big hurry a couple tablespoons of peanut butter in a dish makes a great dip for apples. Better than caramel covered apples any day of the week!

Main Dishes

The real challenge on a gluten free vegan diet is the main course. Snacks and sides are fairly simple as you can always choose from a variety of in season fruits and vegetables. Here are a few main dishes you can experiment with.

Vegetables and Rice

This is a delicious filling main dish and keeping it gluten free and vegan friendly couldn't be simpler.

2 cups uncooked rice
2 medium onions
2 carrots
2 tomatoes or 14 oz. can of stewed tomatoes
3 whole cloves of garlic
3 celery stalks (no leaves)
1 bay leaf (optional)
Salt and pepper to taste
Sit rice and tomatoes aside, separately. Begin preparations by chopping onions, carrots and celery into medium to large chunks. Place all vegetables in stock pot

and add enough water to completely cover. Next add garlic, cloves and a dash of salt and pepper. Bring water and vegetables to a boil over high heat, then reduce heat and simmer for 45 minutes to an hour. About half way through add stewed tomatoes to the mix.

When vegetables are soft but not mushy, remove from heat and strain 3-4 cups of broth. Place rice in a medium sized pan, cover with vegetable broth and cook according to type of rice. Serve vegetables on bed of fragrant rice and enjoy!

NOTE: You can add other vegetables as the fancy strikes, potatoes, peas and even corn can create a colorful and tasty dish. You can also alter garlic and onion amounts to suit your personal preferences.

Chickpea Salad

Gluten free and vegan friendly this little salad is chock full of protein and fiber, which means it, is a salad that will stick with you until dinnertime. This makes a perfect light, yet healthy lunch alternative.

2 cups Chickpeas- cooked
1 oz. olive oil
1 large cucumber- sliced
1/3 cup of fresh dill- finely chopped
1 lemon- juice and zest

Place dry chickpeas in a large bowl, completely cover with water and allow to soak overnight. Drain chickpeas, place in a large pot or stock pan and add four cups of water. (Water is always double the amount of chickpeas). Bring to a boil over high heat, reduce temperature and cook for approximately one hour or until chickpeas are done to your personal preference. Place in bowl, top with sliced cucumber and set aside.

Combine dill, lemon juice and zest in a mixing bowl and whisk together, creating a tasty dressing for your chickpea and cucumber salad.

Pasta Marinara

Who doesn't love a big bowl of pasta on occasion? Thankfully, today's gluten free pasta's taste much better than they used to! Remember the days when you could not be sure if you were eating the noodles or the box? No more my friend!

8 oz. dry gluten free vegan pasta
1 cup chopped green bell pepper
1 cup chopped onion
3 cloves garlic- minced
½ cup chopped celery
½ cup chopped carrots
4 tablespoons olive oil
6 oz. tomato paste
14-16 oz. can tomatoes
1-teaspoon dry oregano
1-teaspoon dry basil
½-teaspoon dry thyme
1-teaspoon sugar
½-cup water

Heat oil in a large skillet and cook together until tender carrots, garlic, onion, celery and peppers. Add tomatoes, spices, tomato paste, ½-cup water and sugar. Bring entire mixture to a boil the reduce heat, cover and simmer ½ hour. Stir occasionally, checking for desired consistency.

Follow packaged directions for preparing your particular brand of gluten free pasta. Most pasta is best served al dente. Cook pasta, drain, add marinara sauce and serve. Serves 4-6 people.

Possible Gluten Free Pasta Option:

Gluten free pasta is a bit easier to find than vegan-gluten free pasta! When all else fails you can make your own!

Simple Mexican Stew

If you thought you would have to give up your favorite type of food to stay on a gluten free vegan path, think again. Mexican stew is easy to make and delicious too!

16 oz. cupful brown beans
4 onions
4 potatoes
6 tomatoes
4 Tablespoon sugar
2 cups grape-juice
2-lemon rind
Water
2-teaspoon cumin
1-teaspoon paprika
1-teaspoon chili powder

Soak beans in approximately 10 cups of water for around 12 hours, overnight usually works. Chop vegetables into bite sized chunks. Add all ingredients to stockpot with beans and simmer for about an hour.

Simple Spanish Rice

Just in case you want a little something extra to go with you Mexican stew. Spanish rice is very simple to make, though there are dozens of alternatives to this particular recipe.

½-pound rice
1 can rotel
8 oz. tomato sauce
1-teaspoon ground cumin
½-teaspoon chili powder
½-teaspoon paprika

Cook rice according to package instructions, combine remaining ingredients adjusting spices to your personal preferences. Always strive to keep cumin levels higher than chili powder, unless you want a nice pan of "chili" rice. After adding tomato sauce, rotel and spices warm slightly over low heat, remember to stir this mixture well especially while warming.

NOTE: Do not be afraid to tinker with the spices, if you will remember to keep the cumin levels slightly higher than the chili powder and paprika you will always get a taco like flavor. You can also add some nice fresh corn for added flavor, color and deliciousness!

Vegetable Pot Pie

Do you recall those lovely little pot pies grandma used to pop in the oven when you were little? Enjoy this comfort food all over again with a tasty gluten free vegan alternative. Enjoy the memories of childhood while maintaining your diet.

1 T olive oil
3 carrots peeled
2 stalks celery
1 red bell pepper
1 medium onion, diced
1-cup fresh peas
1 clove minced garlic
2 new potatoes- chopped or diced small
1/2 cup dry white wine
1/2 cup gluten-free flour
2 cups mushroom stock
1-cup non-dairy milk (soy, coconut, almond, etc…)
1 T sage- roughly chopped

Take half a tablespoon of olive oil, place in medium saucepan over high heat. Stir in carrots, celery, bell pepper, garlic, potatoes and onion. Cook over medium high heat for approximately five minutes. Pour in white wine and reduce heat, cook for another 15 minutes. In a separate saucepan, use the other half of the olive oil to sauté your mushrooms.

Combine sautéed mushrooms and other vegetables together, add mushroom stock (vegetable stock works well also), peas and sage. Sprinkle all of the ingredients with gluten free flour. Stir to ensure flour breaks up nicely and add non-dairy milk. Cook over low heat for about 5 minutes, give or take. At this point, you are ready to transfer vegetable mixture to piecrust, shell.

Use the recipe above for gluten free vegan piecrust, make two balls of dough. Roll out and prepare two crusts, one to line the pie pan and the other for the top crust. Bake in a 425 degree oven for 10-15 minutes, reduce oven temperature to 325 and bake approximately one hour, or until crust is a golden brown.

Side Dishes

Potato Rice Balls

Do you want a side dish that will go with nearly any main course? Potato rice balls will do the trick nicely.

One large onion- finely chopped
Four large potatoes
One cup cooked rice
Olive oil

Cook potatoes and onions together until potatoes are mash able. Mash potatoes, mix in pre-cooked rice, season to taste and form into medium sized balls. Cook in large skillet with olive oil until heated through. For added flavor, green bell peppers and garlic make wonderful additions.

Vegan Baked Potato

Have you been wondering if you would ever have another delicious baked potato? If you crave a loaded baked potato covered in butter, cheese and sour cream, you are out of luck. However, if you want a fantastic tasting alternative that is good for you too, try this wonderful recipe.

2-3 medium to large russet potatoes
1 c broccoli florets
1 c cauliflower pieces
1 c carrots- matchstick
2 cloves chopped garlic
1/4 c apple juice, unsweetened
1 T lemon juice or balsamic vinegar
1/2- 1 tsp. lemon pepper
1 tsp. Italian Herb seasoning
Cooking Spray- olive oil preferably

Wash and wrap baking potatoes, place in 400-degree oven. Bake for approximately 20 minutes or until done.

While potatoes cook, combine cauliflower, carrots, broccoli, and garlic together. Spray generously with olive oil cooking spray. Add seasonings and toss with lemon juice and unsweetened apple juice. Place vegetables in a glass-baking dish, and cook on bottom rack of oven for about 40 minutes. Vegetables and potatoes should be fork tender when done.

Remove all from oven, split baked potato and garnish with vegetable mixture. For added pleasure top with a small amount of vegan grated parmesan cheese.

Chestnut Rissoles

Rissoles are a dish not unlike a meat loaf because basically anything goes! These were popular during and immediately after WWII as a way to make food, particularly meat go further. Leftover meats would be mixed with mashed potatoes, carrots, onions or anything that was available, then rolled in flour and fried for a tasty little cake. This is but one gluten free vegan rissole alternative.

1-pound Chestnuts
1 T chopped Parsley
1 T corn flour
1 T water

Cook chestnuts over medium high heat for about 30 minutes. Remove from stove, shell and mash nuts to form a paste. In a separate bowl combine cornmeal and water, mix well. Use the cornmeal mixture to moisten chestnut paste. Form rissole paste into small, rather flat pieces and roll in either vegan flour mixture or extra cornmeal. Fry in your choice of oils and serve.

Polenta and Corn

There are so many ways to prepare and use polenta; it has even been used as a noodle substitute for vegan lasagna! For today's busy families however, simpler is often best particularly when it comes to gluten free vegan diets.

2 c water
2 c unsweetened soymilk
1 tsp. salt
1 c cornmeal
1 T vegan buttery spread (earth balance is a good choice)
1/3 c unflavored, gluten-free soy creamer
2 tablespoons yeast (not brewer's yeast!)
1 1/2 c fresh corn

In a medium saucepan combine water, salt, and soymilk over medium heat, bring to a boil. Carefully whisk in cornmeal mixture and reduce heat. Stir constantly to remove lumps and prevent scorching, (about two minutes). Add vegan butter spread stirring until mixture is nice and creamy. Cook about 20 minutes, adding water if mix becomes to dry or thick.

When polenta has reached desired consistency stir in corn, yeast and soy creamer. You may need to cook mixture over low heat for a few more minutes after adding the last few ingredients.

Desserts

Zucchini Banana Spice Cake

Spice cake like mom used to make? On a gluten free vegan diet? Yes, yes you can! All it takes is a few minor alterations and you have a great desert you can enjoy morning, noon or night.

1 Pound Zucchini- peeled and grated (approximately 3 cups)
16 oz. flaked coconut
16 oz. walnuts- ground
12 tablespoons pureed banana
1 ½-cup tapioca starch flour
1 ½ cup white rice flour (mixing the two prevents a grainy texture)
1-teaspoon baking powder
1-teaspoon baking soda
2 teaspoons vanilla
2 ½ cups sugar
1 teaspoon of salt
Preheat oven 350°

Mix together coconut, walnuts and zucchini then set aside. Beat together pureed bananas, vanilla and oil in large mixing bowl. Beat in sugar and gradually add remaining dry ingredients, beating the mixture well. Add zucchini mixture, gently mix and pour into prepared cake pan/pans. (2-10 inch pans work well) Bake for 35-45 minutes. Allow to cool and frost to taste.

Creamy Apple Tapioca

An apple a day keeps the doctor away, and is there any better way to preserve your health? It may not be an apple fritter or cobbler, but it is quite tasty anyway.

1/2 cup tapioca
2-5 apples - approximately a pound
2 cups water
Sugar to taste
Lemon peel- grated yellow side
1 tsp. cinnamon (optional)

Preparations for this sweet dish begin the night before! Soak tapioca in 2 cups of water overnight. Peel, core and slice apples in quarters. In a medium sauce pan cook apples over medium low heat until they are nice and tender. Next, place them in a pie pan, sprinkle with sugar, grated part of lemon peel, and cinnamon (if you like). Finally mix in tapioca and water and bake for about an hour at 350 degrees. Remove from oven, serve chilled.

Strawberries in Cherry Syrup

If you are counting calories, you might want to skip this particular recipe! Nevertheless, if you do by chance have a skip day coming, try your hand at this delectable treat.

1-pound Strawberries
1-pound Cherries
2 C water
2 C granulated sugar

If you want to go really old school with this recipe, dust off your mortar and pestle! Start by grinding the cherries, pit and all, into a pasty substance. Place crushed cherries, water and sugar into a medium saucepan. Boil uncovered for one hour.

Strain cherry syrup into a smaller saucepan and reduce over medium heat until syrup begins to thicken. Remove from heat add strawberries to syrup and stir or shake around to thoroughly cover. Place strawberries on serving platter, return syrup to stove and cook for a few more minutes to thicken further. Drizzle remaining sauce over strawberries, allow to cool and enjoy!

Banana Nut Bread

An all-time favorite comfort food! If you thought you were going to have to give it up on your gluten free vegan diet, you will be very happy to find this recipe.

2 cups gluten-free all-purpose baking flour
1-teaspoon baking soda
1/4 teaspoon salt
1/2 cup soymilk
2 cups mashed ripe bananas (4-5 medium)
3/4 cup sugar
1/4 cup brown sugar
1/2 cup unsweetened applesauce
1/3 cup canola oil
1/2 tsp. cinnamon
1-teaspoon vanilla extract
2 T Maple Syrup

First, mix all dry ingredients in a mixing bowl, set aside.

Combine wet ingredients, mix well and add to dry ingredients.

Place dough in two 8x4 inch loaf pans and bake at 350 degrees for approximately 45 minutes. Loafs tend to be a bit crumbly so allow to cool for several minutes before removing from loaf pans. Your friends will never know this is a gluten free vegan recipe!

Vegan Gluten Free Chocolate Chip Cookies

As you know, most chocolate chips are not on the vegan approved grocery list so you may have despaired ever smelling the chocolate goodness that is the chocolate chip cookie. Rest assured there is a gluten free vegan alternative.

1/2 C Tapioca Starch
1/2 C brown rice flour
1/2 C sorghum flour
1/2 C potato starch
1/2 C Granulated sugar
1/2 teaspoon xanthan gum
1/2 teaspoon baking soda
1/2 teaspoon salt
1/2 C grape seed oil
3/4 C pure maple syrup
2 teaspoons vanilla
1/2-3/4 cup vegan chocolate chips

Mix together dry ingredients in a medium mixing bowl. Next stir in vanilla, oil and maple syrup. You can mix ingredients by hand or use a mechanical mixer on a medium setting. Mixture will be slightly thin but add in chocolate chips and allow to stand for about 10 minutes.

It will thicken up.

Drop cookie dough on prepared baking sheets by the tablespoon and bake for around 10 minutes. Cookies should look a bit doughy and underdone. Allow to cool on the baking sheet for a few minutes, (cookies will continue to cook for a bit after coming out of the oven.)

Soups

Sometimes nothing satisfies like a warm bowl of tasty soup. If you are tired of trying to find a good gluten free vegan soup from the canned varieties in your local store, here are a few homemade soups to add to your recipe box.

Gluten Free Vegan Tomato Soup

Are you feeling a bit under the weather? Perhaps you just want something that is filling but light on the stomach at the same time. Gluten free vegan tomato soup sounds like the perfect solution.

2 cans Stewed Tomatoes
1 large carrot.
1 large turnip.
1 large onion.
2 1/4 cups of water.
3 ounces vegan butter.
1-tablespoon sago.
2 teaspoons salt.

1 tsp. dried tarragon
1-tablespoon lemon juice
Pepper to taste

Dice onion, carrot, and turnip. In a medium saucepan heat half vegan, butter sauté gently. Add pepper, salt and water to mix and boil gently. Once vegetables are quite tender pour in stewed tomatoes, salt to taste and other half of vegan butter. Simmer all ingredients together with tarragon, lemon juice and pepper for approximately 60 minutes or until vegetables are thoroughly cooked. Allow mixture to cool slightly then puree until smooth and enjoy.

Hearty Mexican Soup

Here is a favorite that is a little heartier than your traditional soup!

1 can chili beans
1 can pinto beans
½ C onion- finely chopped
1 can stewed tomatoes (diced works as well)
2 tsp. ground cumin
1 tsp. chili powder
1 tsp. paprika
Garlic powder to taste
1 ½ C water

Bring all ingredients to a boil in a medium saucepan. Reduce heat and simmer for 15-20 minutes. Serve with your favorite gluten free vegan chips, sour cream and vegan cheese!

Reduce water to increase consistency and this makes a great filler for corn tortilla. One recipe that doubles as two meals.

Potato, Squash and Apple Soup

You might be a little ambiguous about adding apples to a vegetable soup recipe, but give it a chance. This might just become your favorite cold weather concoction.

1/2 butternut squash
1 medium red potatoes
2 or more garlic cloves- minced
1 green apples, peeled and chopped
Salt and pepper to taste
1-2 sprigs of fresh thyme (1/2 tsp. of dried can be substituted)
Olive oil
2 cups of vegetable stock

Prepare squash and potatoes. Peel, de-seed squash and cut both into bite-sized cubes. Next peel, core and quarter green apple. Set aside.

Sauté minced garlic with olive oil in a medium sized stockpot. Cook until golden. Add vegetables and apple to your sautéed garlic and cook for a few minutes. (2-5) Next add vegetable stock, reduce heat and allow soup to simmer until potatoes and squash are fork tender.

French Cabbage Soup

Who said vegan and gluten free recipes had to be all-American? Take the French cabbage soup out for a test drive today!

3 carrots
1 turnip
1 leek
2 sticks celery
1/2 cabbage
1 bay leaf
2 whole cloves
5 peppercorns
12 C. water.

Peel and dice carrots and turnips, dice celery, slice the leek and shred the 1/2 head of cabbage.

Place all ingredients together in a large stockpot. Bring water and vegetables to a boil and then reduce heat. Allow soup to simmer on low for 2-3 hours. At the end of the day, you have a delicious, healthy soup.

Raw Foods, Seasonal Favorites and Drinks

You might think adding another diet category to a gluten free vegan lifestyle would be unnecessarily difficult, but when that category is raw food, it actually makes a lot of sense. Gluten free and vegan fit very nicely with a raw food diet, and gives you a few more recipe alternatives.

Pineapple Banana Drink

1 C fresh banana
1 C fresh pineapple
2 C spinach
1/2 C water
2-3 regular ice cubes
Place all ingredients in a blender and process on high speeds until contents are smooth. You can ditch the ice by using frozen produce instead. You should know this drink will be quite green, thanks to the spinach!

Bacon- Sort Of!

Do you ever get a hankering for some good old-fashioned bacon? What if you could achieve the flavor and texture without betraying your vegan lifestyle? Enter eggplant bacon!

1 lb. eggplant
4 TBS gluten free soy sauce
1 tsp. liquid smoke

Create a marinade from the gluten free soy sauce and liquid smoke, set aside. Cut your eggplant in to small strips, about 1/8 inch to be exact. Place eggplant strips in marinade, making sure each piece is covered well. Allow vegetable to soak for at least a couple of hours.

At this point you have a couple of alternatives, you can use a dehydrator set on 116 for approximately 12 hours or bake your eggplant bacon. Pre-heat oven to 425 degrees and bake for 8-10 minutes turning once and baking for another 2-4 minutes. The result is a bacon alternative that you can eat alone or as a topping for your favorite dish. (Perhaps a gluten free vegan baked potato?)

"Eggnog"

Have you always enjoyed the holidays and in particular eggnog? You will probably be hard pressed to find a good tasting vegan eggnog, so why not make your own?

1/2 cup cashews
1/2 cup macadamia nuts
2 cups water
Sea salt to taste
6 tbs. agave nectar
Pinch of nutmeg

In your trusty blender process, all ingredients until they are relatively smooth. Remove any small particles of nuts by running your mixture through a cheesecloth or something similar. Serve slightly chilled and enjoy.

Vegan Cocoa

Another seasonal favorite that many hate to mark off their list is hot chocolate or cocoa. Good news, you do not have to!

1 C almond milk
1 1/2 T cocoa powder (unsweetened of course)
2 tsp. sugar

In a small saucepan, cook almond milk until it is steaming hot, but not boiling. Stir in sugar and cocoa mix, add a stick of cinnamon on the side and you are ready to settle in on any chilly evening.

Holiday Favorite Pumpkin Pie

1 16 oz. can pumpkin
½ C granulated sugar
¼ C brown sugar
1 C soy milk (almond is good too)
1 tsp. vanilla
¼ tsp. nutmeg
¼ tsp. allspice
½ tsp. cinnamon
1 gluten free pie crust (purchased or made from recipe above)

Blend all ingredients in a medium mixing bowl with an electric hand mixer on low speeds. Mix for 3-4 minutes. Pour mixture into gluten free vegan pie shells, insert into 425-degree oven for 15 minutes. Turn down oven to 350 degrees and bake for about 45 minutes. Allow dish to cool before consuming.

Gluten Free Vegan Staples for the Pantry

Now that you have made the decision to change your life, what do you need to do first? If you have always consumed a traditional diet, you may want to start slowly by choosing a few items to replace as you learn new recipes. You have several alternative items to work with, which means it could get expensive quickly. Choose one or two from each category to begin your transition to a healthier lifestyle.

- Oils
- Extra virgin olive oil
- Saffron Oil
- Coconut oil
- Sunflower oil
- Beans
- Pinto
- Navy
- Kidney
- Black-eyed Peas
- (pretty much any dried bean is good for a gluten free vegan diet)

- Whole Grain Flour
- Cornmeal
- Quinoa
- Spelt
- Rice flour
- Herbs and Spices

This is another category where pretty much anything goes, however two come to mind as particularly useful.

Italian Seasoning
Curry powder

Finally-

Fruits, vegetables and rice tend to be fantastic starter foods for a gluten free vegan diet. There are so many dishes you can create with these ingredients and some imagination!

Health Concerns of a Vegan Gluten Free Diet

The general consensus for the health of a gluten free vegan diet is that it is good, provided you are willing to supplement your diet to make up for a few key vitamins and minerals that will be lacking. By excluding both dairy and meat products from your diet you lose several key minerals and vitamins. If you want to be successful and healthy with this type of restrictive diet, here are a few of the supplements you will need to consume.

Vitamin B-12

Vitamin B-12 is very important to the healthy function of the human body. B-12 is necessary for the production of red blood cells, which carry much needed oxygen throughout the body. Deficiencies in this vitamin can lead to lethargy and weakness.

Foods rich in B-12 include:
Beef liver
Clams
Rainbow trout

Eggs
Chicken breast

You cannot get enough vitamin B-12 from your diet when you follow a gluten free vegan lifestyle. Thankfully, there are supplements on the market to help you make up for the short fall in your daily diet.

Iron

Another building block of blood is iron, which is typically found in adequate levels if you eat a varied diet. Vegans and vegetarians, however, have such a limited diet it is difficult to get adequate amounts from food alone since the richest sources are items such as:

Calf liver
Cooked oysters
Cuttlefish
Octopus
Beef heart
Various organ meats

You will probably here a lot of people tout the iron levels of soybeans, lentils, spinach and various other vegetables but you should know these are two different types of iron. Meat based iron is known as Heme-iron while plant based is non-heme. The major difference in the two is absorption rates, heme iron absorbs much more readily than non-heme varieties. Therefore, if you are vegan or vegetarian you should make it a point to consume more iron rich vegetables such as kale, broccoli and legumes (beans).

Omega-3 Fatty Acids

The loss of eggs and fish from your diet leave you at risk for omega-3 deficiencies. Cold water fish such as sardines and mackerel are two of the best sources of this essential nutrient. However, walnuts, flaxseed oil, soybeans and canola oil are great sources as well. Many people opt for fish oil capsules as a supplement, but that may not sit well with your vegan lifestyle.

Calcium

Your bones and teeth depend on adequate calcium, without it, you could face tooth loss and early onset osteoporosis or worse. Most people do not realize that calcium deficiency can leave you vulnerable to hypertension, abnormal heartbeat and in severe cases convulsions!

Calcium also plays a major role in many other functions of the human body such as hormone secretion, nerve transmission, muscle stimulation and so much more. Calcium deficiency can lead to brittle nails; hair loss, heart arrhythmia, anxiety and severe irritation just to name a few.

Since milk, cheese and fish are off the menu it is important that you consume a diet high in plant-based calcium and take vitamin D supplements. Vitamin D is necessary for calcium absorption and is another vitamin taken off the menu with the vegan gluten free diet.

Gluten Free Concerns

In most cases there are no real risks with a gluten free diet, in fact the human body does not absorb gluten but passes it through the digestive system. The biggest concern with this type of limiting diet is nutrition. As with a vegan diet, there are a few essential vitamins and minerals you will be missing out on, and since many people replace, breads with higher calorie nuts you could theoretically gain weight on a gluten free diet.

If you feel you may have a gluten sensitivity or celiac

disease it is important that you talk to your medical professional. Ask him or her to perform the necessary blood test to confirm your suspicions, before you begin a specialized diet. Celiac disease symptoms are relatively common and similar to several other ailments, so you may have to ask for the test specifically as many doctors do not think to perform it as a routine test.

Gluten Free Vegan Conclusion

Is it possible to lead a gluten free vegan life? A few years ago, the outlook would have been grim but thanks to the wide variety of gluten free and vegan friendly products on the market today it has never been easier. More importantly, it is now possible to follow this type of diet and still be able to consume great tasting dishes. There are a few concerns and questions that come up when considering a radical change, here are a few of the most common.

Vegan FAQ's

Is a vegan diet healthy?

According to the American Dietetic Association, there is no reason a vegetarian or vegan diet cannot provide a nutritional alternative. That being said, your diet needs to be well planned so that all your essential vitamins, minerals and fatty acids are accounted for, as mentioned above.

How difficult is it to go vegan?

Depending on how rigidly you plan to adhere to the vegan principles, it can be very difficult at first. The key to making this type of transition is to start slowly, making small changes. Any step toward an animal friendly existence is a good one.

Is a vegan diet expensive?

Again, this depends a lot on your approach. Purchasing the majority of your diet in the form of pre-packaged vegan alternatives can get quite expensive. However, if you compare the cost of vegetables, beans and other staple vegan items with the rising costs of meat you may find the vegan diet is quite a bit cheaper.

Gluten Free FAQ's

What foods can I eat?

It is actually easier to discuss what you should avoid. Any foods that contain wheat, rye and barley are out of the question. The key is to learn which items on an ingredient list are derived from one of the above. For example malt, triticale and malt vinegar are all derived from items on the banned list.

Why are oats such a big deal?

Pure oats are gluten free and perfectly acceptable on a gluten free diet. However, until recently commercially packaged oats were often exposed to cross contamination from wheat, rye or barley. Read your labels carefully, particularly if you are a celiac sufferer.

Is celiac disease really that bad?

Over time and left untreated celiac disease can cause a variety of health problems. Since the villi in the intestine are continually destroyed it becomes harder and harder for the body to get the nutrition it needs. This can lead to brittle bones, skin conditions, anemia and other ailments.

Should you start a gluten free vegan diet today? Whether you suffer celiac disease or simply want a diet plan that puts you on the right track to losing weight and feeling better this could be the answer for you.

Create a plan for putting this diet in place, after all if you have always lived a traditional lifestyle it can be quite a shock to just empty the pantry and refrigerator and start on what may seem like a foreign diet.

Baby Steps

In the beginning, the easiest transition will be away from meat products. Slowly begin phasing out your favorite meat dishes for healthier vegetarian options. This is a good time to begin experimenting with tofu and different ways to create mock meat dishes. Silken tofu is a good option and can be processed to resemble ground beef for Italian dishes.

CAUTION: If you do opt for vegan meat alternatives found in the grocery store you should read the labels carefully. Many of these products contain wheat, rye or barley and are not appropriate for a gluten free diet.

Next, you could switch your whole, two percent or skim milk for a soy or nut milk alternative. There are several commercially produced non-dairy milks on the shelves today thanks to the number of people who are lactose intolerant. Do not be afraid to try different brands and types of milk until you find one that suits your taste buds.

Keep it Simple

Vegan and gluten free recipes are very easy to find, however not all of them are simple. When you are first starting out keep it simple. Complicated recipes can result in at best a tasteless dish and at worst something, you would not feed your dog! This could derail your entire plan for a gluten free vegan diet, so opt for easy to make recipes that do not contain a large number of bizarre ingredients or spices.

Substitute

Do you have some favorite recipes you would really hate to give up on? Work on making vegan and gluten free substitutions. While this might seem like a daunting task at first, you will soon discover which binding agents work best in each type of recipe and which vegetables can be substituted for meat or gluten based products.

NOTE: This task is not for the faint at heart or those who are easily discouraged. Be prepared to throw away and laugh at some of your more epic failures. It is through this process you will grow and become a more knowledgeable cook and successful vegan.

Gluten Free Vegan -- In Summary

A gluten free vegan diet may not sound like the easiest path in the world to take, but when your health is on the line, it is definitely worth the trouble. Plan your progress, choose nutrient high foods and take the appropriate supplements when necessary. Talk to your medical professional about monitoring for things like calcium, B-12, iron and magnesium.

Section 2: Paleolithic Cookbook

The standard western diet may be hurting or killing your body in so many ways, that it can be difficult to keep up with all of the health reports related to unhealthy eating. The Paleolithic diet has been popularly known for many decades, however history seems to show that early human ancestors were living on this "diet" was around 200,000 years ago! Humans were introduced into farming approximately 10,000 years producing a heavy growth grains, bread, pasta, starchy foods and processed foods. However, evidence suggests that evolution is slow to adapt to new types of food that the body may not be used to. This is why the foods including (modern) bread, grease, and processed foods are hard for humans to move on from and onto a healthier lifestyle.

What is Paleo?

The paleo lifestyle tries to follow the diet of those from ancient times of indigenous people and is referred to as the "Paleolithic Diet" as it is from the Stone Age or Paleolithic Age era. The paleo diet has additional names it is referred to including, "Stone Age Diet", "Hunter-Gatherer Diet", or the "Cave Man Diet". The Paleolithic diet offers a plethora of health benefits for those who have given it a try. The paleo diet isn't another fad diet as it has been a way of eating thousands of years and it is a healthier option for people to take. Anthropologists have found that tribal people who have only been on the paleo diet are slimmer, stronger and healthier compared to those who aren't on the diet. These people do not suffer with cavities, dental problems, and have straight teeth. They also have perfect eyesight, rarely battle with arthritis, diabetes, obesity, heart disease, stroke, depression, cancer, and hypertension and schizophrenia disorders. There are approximately 84 tribes of hunter-gatherers left in this world who eat a Paleolithic diet. These people get daily adequate exercise which also helps them to stay healthy too. The tribal people have never evolved further like current civilization has done. The paleo diet is an advanced nutritional plan using wild plants and animals of different species. This diet has been around for over 2.5 million years however it ended 10,000 years ago when agriculture was developed. The Paleolithic diet theory introduced dieters with features of holistic and, comprehensive dietary combined together.

Why Go the Paleolithic Diet Route?

The paleo diet route should provide everything that the body needs to function properly. The primary dietary components are all covered, such as vitamins, phytosterols, proteins, fats, carbohydrates, and antioxidants. This diet is needed as it is programmed within our genes to eat these types of foods and discard foods that do not fit within the paleo diet.

Indigenous cultures that are around in this present day still eat the same diet of foods they have eaten for centuries have been considered primitive for not changing their diets. Instead these hunter-gatherers eat the foods that are in their area don't suffer what modern eaters suffer with today. Anthropologists has studied and compared these people with modernized people and they found that the results in association between diet and disease is completely clear that diseases such as diabetes, heart disease, cancer, arthritis and many other diseases were rarely found among the hunter gatherers.

Many dieters found that, after eating Paleo for three weeks:

- BMI dropped by about 0.8
- Average weight loss was around 5 pounds
- Blood pressure fell by an average of three mmHg
- Increase in antioxidants
- Healthier potassium-sodium balance
- Levels of plasminogen activator inhibitor (blood thickening agent) dropped by 72%.

Benefits of the Paleo Lifestyle

The top benefit of the Paleo diet are eating foods that are naturally high in fiber. Fiber helps to reduce constipation, lower cholesterol, and lowers risks of diabetes and coronary heart disease. The paleo diet focuses on helping people lose weight with eating foods that were available during the Paleolithic era. These foods consist of meat, eggs, vegetables, roots, fish, mushrooms and berries. Our bodies are designed to handle foods loaded in high protein, and low carbohydrates however we are not genetically ready to handle low protein and high carb diets during these modern times. Eating a natural diet instead of a diet filled with processed foods, sugar-filled, and grain products.

The paleo diet offers the body a higher proportion of fat compared to the average Western diet. This higher proportion gives the body an additional health benefit of providing more energy and helps the body perform better. The fat found in modern diets is primarily unhealthy, consisting of a lot of trans fats. The quality of fat a body needs to consist of fat soluble nutrients including vitamins A, D, E, and K and the CoQ10 (coenzyme) can't be absorbed without the presence of fat. All of these vitamins are very important for the body and avoiding nutrient deficiencies.
Omega-3's provides many benefits for the body such as helping to increase brain size, and forming brain tissue. The omega-3 fatty acids are essential in supporting biochemical processes, creating membranes in cells which keep tissues healthy and maintaining the body's metabolism. It not only improves physical health but also improves mental health, build immune system, cardiovascular strength, and healthy digestion.

Paleo Food Types

Foods to eat

The Paleo diets come into different types of restrictions depending on the dieter's preferences. The basic paleo diet consists of eating foods that are as close to nature or as natural as possible. These foods include:

- Meats – lean beef, chuck steak, lean veal, long broil, top sirloin, chicken, fish, pork, seafood, etc.
- Other Meat – venison, alligator, bison, reindeer, rabbit, pheasant, wild turkey, wild boar, goal, rattlesnake, emu, caribou, etc.
- Vegetables -
- Fruits
- Nuts & seeds
- Seed oils – olive, avocado, palm, coconut, almond, walnut, pecan, macadamia, hazelnut)
- Water
- Coffee and tea - drink the coffee black or with unsweetened almond milk

Foods to avoid

- Grains – barley, oats, rice, wheat, maize, rye, wild rice, millet, corn, etc.
- Grain-like Seeds – buckwheat, quinoa, amaranth
- Sugar – soft drinks, fruit drinks, candy, honey
- Legumes – all beans, lentils, miso, etc
- Dairy – butter, cheese, ice cream, milk, yogurt, creamer
- Any processed foods

Paleo Confusion

How to know if a food type adheres to the paleo plan.

There are many continuous ongoing debates on whether a certain food type adheres to the paleo plan as the diet focuses on what the first people ate before farming began. However, research is being done to find out if the first people ate potatoes. However, most speculate they did. The confusion comes from certain foods that can't really be classified as Paleo or not, like honey, oats or potato. The truth is, that the paleo diet plan isn't completely cut and dry. Saying that, most of the foods listed as paleo provide enough variety and satiety to continue with, without feeling like "cheating".

Paleo Food List

All of the following foods are paleo friendly to eat.

- Protein
- Eggs
- Fish
    - bass
    - cod
    - mackerel
    - grouper
    - halibut
    - herring
    - red snapper
    - salmon

- Lean Beef and lean cuts
    - Steaks – flank and chuck
      Lean hamburger beef
    - Veal
    - Sirloin

- Lean Lamb
    - lamb chops and loin

- Lean Poultry
    - Chicken, hen and turkey breast

- Other Meats
    - bison – ostrich
    - elk - squab
    - alligator - goat
    - bear - goose
    - kangaroo - caribou
    - pheasant - rattlesnake
    - rabbit –quail
    - reindeer - emu
    - turtle – wild turkey
    - wild boar - venison

- Shellfish
    - crab - clams
    - abalone - crayfish
    - lobster – shrimp
    - scallops - oysters
    - mussels

- Fats
    - Brazil nuts - almonds
    - Avocado - coconut
    - cashews – flaxseed oil
    - coconut oil
    - chestnuts

- Cold pressed nuts and seeds
    - walnuts
    - pecans pumpkin seeds
    - pistachios
    - pine nuts

- sunflower seeds
- sesame seeds

- Vegetables
    - cauliflower - celery
    - artichoke - asparagus
    - beet greens
    - beets - bell pepper
    - broccoli
    - Kale - Brussels sprouts
    - cabbage – carrots - tomato
    - endive - green onion
    - Kohlrabi - watercress
    - collards - cucumber
    - lettuce - mushroom
    - mustard greens
    - onions - parsley
    - parsnip - peppers
    - pumpkin - rutabaga
    - radish - seaweed
    - spinach - tomatillos
    - Swiss chard – squash
    - turnips and turnip greens

- Fruits
    - apple - apricot
    - banana - blackberry
    - boysenberry - papaya
    - cantaloupe - cassava melon
    - cherimoya - cherries
    - cranberry - figs

- gooseberry - grapefruit
- grapes - guava
- honeydew -lychee
- lemon - lime
- kiwi –orange -mango
- nectarine -
- passion fruit -plums
- peaches - pears
- persimmon - pineapple
- pomegranate - strawberry
- raspberry – tangerine
- star fruit - watermelon
- tangerine
- rhubarb

Sample Daily Meal Plan for Beginners

It can be difficult coming up with an original menu plan and easily eat something that is not Paleo related. The best option is to create a menu plan that will help you to make some good food choices and consistently stay on your Paleo diet. Create a meal plan that will last for a week or two so if possible purchase at least two weeks worth of food. Keep in mind that it's okay you can skip a meal whenever you want as the Paleo diet isn't about eating three meals a day. In this sample menu day plan there are **three** meals and a snack added providing you with enough options to work and play around with it.

Sample Menu Day Plan:

	Breakfast	Lunch	Dinner
Monday	Berries with coconut milk and mixed nuts	Broccoli and Pine Nut Soup	Meatballs with Crunchy Sweet Potato Chips
Tuesday	Scrambled Eggs with Mushroom	Cucumber Hot Dogs	Pumpkin and Chicken Curry
Wednesday	Salmon and Zucchini Fritters	Roast Vegetables in Orange and Rosemary	Chicken with Macadamia Topping
Thursday	Mushroom and Meat Omelet	Dory with Beetroot Salad	Lamb Chops
Friday	Lemon Pancakes	Moroccan Lamb with Squash	Chicken and Egg Salad with Almond Sautée Sauce

Eating Paleo in Day to Day Life

Restaurants and Eating Out

Paleo dieters need to find paleo food friendly restaurants and eateries that cater specifically to their diet. There has been a slow trickle of restaurants available catering to natural and raw foods for health conscious people. Avoid leaving your Paleo diet up to chance as the failure rates are high when that is done. Instead look into planning ahead by preparing a list of Paleo-friendly restaurants near your home and work. However, keep in mind that your social life is completely different compared to your Paleo ancestors so there will be a trade off of some sort involved. So look into minimizing the damage and try to find more desirable options on the menu and then tighten up on your diet for the next several days. Your ancestors they didn't have temptations all around them to pull them off of their diet however they didn't consider the Paleo diet as a diet but as a means of survival.

While out in restaurants, tell the waiter you have a gluten allergy and that includes any grains. Be serious about the topic and they will know to take it seriously and make sure that nothing has touched a non-paleo food or product. Ask for your meal to be cooked with olive oil.

Social Eating

When out with friends do let them know that you won't accept any bad foods. They should know about your diet beforehand so that it will not be a surprise. This is especially important if you dealing with an autoimmune disease or a digestive problem, or are trying to lose weight. Bringing some food of your own will also help to alleviate any issues that may arise. Allow your friends to taste the food you're eating and it will give you an added topic to discuss with your friends.

Food Preparation

Food meal planning helps with knowing what to prepare and eat. The sample meal planner in this book helps in providing ideas and deciding on the best options. Preparing your meals ahead of time instead of cooking daily is a timesaver.

Meal Frequency and Amounts

A person should in general eat when they are hungry, however eating at least 3-4 times a day is a good way to go. It all depends on what you feel fits your overall needs and schedule. The idea on the amount of food to consume meets closer to the FDA's RDI (Recommended Daily Intake) measurements. For protein, individuals on a 2000 calorie diet may need approximately 50% of protein.

Recipe Ideas

Breakfast

Mushroom and Pine Nuts Scrambled Eggs

Ingredients

3 eggs
2 teaspoons of finely chopped onions
2 tablespoons of finely chopped chives
1 cup of slice mushrooms
1 tbsp of oil
1 tablespoon of pine nuts
Salt and pepper

Instructions

Place the oil in the frying pan on medium heat and fry the onions for at least 3-4 minutes until they are browned lightly then remove the mushrooms from the pan.

In a bowl whisk the eggs then pour it into the frying pan while constantly stirring the eggs.

Add the chives when the eggs are almost cooked, allow it to cook for another minute or until the eggs are finally cooked.

Add in salt and pepper for flavor, then turn off heat and add in mushrooms, and pine nuts before serving.

Salmon and Zucchini Fritters

Ingredients

1 ½ cups of almond meal
2 eggs
100g of thinly sliced smoked salmon
1 tbsp chopped dill
2 roughly grated large zucchini with the liquid removed
Salt and pepper
1 tablespoon of oil

Instructions:

Combine the eggs and almond meal in a medium bowl, whisking both together until it is smooth.

Stir in the smoked salmon, dill, salt and pepper, and zucchini.

Place the oil in the frying pan over medium heat.

Spoon in approximately 1 tablespoonful of the smoked salmon combination into the frying pan. Make sure to allow it enough room for it to spread.

Fry the mixture for about 2-3 minutes on each side until completely cooked with a golden brown look.

Drain the fritter on either some absorbent paper or a paper towel.

Repeat the same process and add oil to the pan between each batch in order for it to cook properly.

Serve with a delicious green salad such as an arugula green salad.

Lemon Pancakes

2 eggs
1 tbsp of apple sauce
2 tbsp of lemon juice
1/3 cups of almond butter
1 tbsp of coconut oil

Instructions:

Combine all of the ingredients except for the coconut oil into a bowl.

Heat the coconut oil in medium heat in a frying pan. Spoon the pancake mixture into the frying pan.

Fry the pancake for about 1 minute before flipping it over to the other side. Cook for 1 minute on the other side. Serve pancakes and enjoy.

Lunch Recipes

Dory Fillet with Beetroot Salad

Ingredients for the fish:

2 dory fillets
Lemon juice
Salt and pepper

Ingredients for salad:

½ small beetroot – diced finely
½ medium tomato – diced finely
1 cup finely chopped lettuce
5 chopped walnuts
Lemon juice

Instructions:

Preheat oven to 350°F degrees Fahrenheit.

Place the dory fillets in an oven tray and sprinkle it with salt, pepper and lemon juice.

Bake the fish in over for approximately 10-15 minutes.

For the salad, place all of the salad ingredients into a bowl combining them well and add in the lemon juice to taste. Serve the salad with fish and enjoy.

Cucumber Hot Dogs

Ingredients:

4 small sausages
4 small cucumbers
Tomato sauce (optional)

Instructions:

Preheat the grill medium/high heat.
Grill the sausages for about 6-8 minutes or until they are cooked thoroughly.

For the cucumber, cut the ends off the cucumbers and use a small knife or butter knife to remove the seeds by twisting the knife around in circles.

Place a hot sausage in the hollow part of the cucumber and serve with tomato sauce.

Dinner Recipes

Chicken Curry with Pumpkin

Ingredients

5 cups of diced pumpkin
Sliced 2 chicken breasts
2 tablespoons of olive oil
1 diced onion
2 finely chopped up garlic cloves
2 tablespoons of ground ginger
1 tablespoons of ground turmeric
2 tablespoons of ground coriander
2 tablespoons of ground cumin
Vegetable stock 1 ½ cups
1 small fresh heap of coriander, chopped
Add in a dash of salt.

Instructions

Put the diced onion and garlic into a pan, fry with the oil for at least 2-3 minutes on medium heat setting. Add in the sliced chicken and cook consistently stirring for about 10-11 minutes or until chicken has cooked thoroughly becoming white.

Add in the diced pumpkin, turmeric, ginger, cumin, and coriander. Stirring for at least 1 minute.

Add in the vegetable stock and allow it to simmer for approximately 15 minutes on low heat. Add in the chopped coriander, cover the pan and cook for about 2 minutes.

Add a dash of salt to taste.

Sides

Soups and Salads

Broccoli and Pine Nut Soup

Ingredients

1 diced onion
1 tablespoon of oil
3 cups of broccoli
3 cups of vegetable stock or chicken stock
¼ cup of pine nuts

Instructions:

Put the oil and diced onions in a large pan on medium heat until the onions are lightly browned.

Add in the stock and broccoli to the pan and let it simmer for approximately 10-15 minutes or until the broccoli has softened. Let the broccoli cool slightly.

Place the broccoli and stock into a food processor or use an electric blender if you don't own a food processor to create a smoother texture.

Heat the soup and serve.

Roast Vegetables in Orange and Rosemary

(Serves 4-6)

2 cups of diced pumpkin
2 tbsp of olive oil
2 cups of diced sweet potato
1 cup of diced carrots
1 juiced orange
6 tbsp of fresh rosemary leaves
2 finely chopped garlic cloves
Salt and pepper

Instructions

Pre-heat a fan-forced oven to 400 degrees Fahrenheit.

Combine all of the ingredients together and place into an oven proof dish
Bake in oven for 15 minutes. Remove from the oven and stir well to cover the vegetables in the orange liquid then return back to the oven for another 10-15 minutes or until the vegetables are tender.

Meats

Crunchy Sweet Potato Chips with Meatballs

Ingredients

Mince meat - 250g
Almond meal - 1/3 cup
Baby spinach – 3 cups
Tomato paste – approximately 25g
2 tablespoons of fresh sage
1 medium sweet potato
Olive oil
Salt to taste

Instructions

Preheat the oven to 350 degrees Fahrenheit.

Placing the spinach in a bowl, cover it with boiling water. Cook spinach for 2 minutes before draining out as much liquid as possible from the spinach. Chop the spinach.

Place the mince meat, chopped spinach, almond meal,

dash of salt, sage, and tomato paste. Combine the entire ingredients well.

Heat the frying pan to handle deep frying and peel the sweet potato with a vegetable peeler into ribbons. Place a handful of the sweet potato ribbons into the frying pan for about 2 minutes. Allow them to brown slightly. Remove the cooked sweet potato ribbons and place on a plate with a paper towel on it to drain remaining oil.

Roll the mixture into 2.5cm size balls and place them on a baking tray lined with baking paper.

Bake in the oven for 10-15 minutes or until browned and cooked thoroughly.

On a plate place the meatballs with the sweet potato ribbons top of them.

Peppered Steak

Ingredients

4 - 100g rump steaks
Crushed peppercorns 4 tablespoons
1 beaten egg
1 tbsp oil

Instructions

Immerse the steak into the egg mixture, and then cover with crushed peppercorns.

Put the steak into pan or barbeque grill with some oil to grease. Fry on high setting for about 30 seconds on each side, then reduce down the heat and cook until steak is cooked tenderly.

Eat with boiled vegetables and/or crispy green salad.

Paprika Lamb

Ingredients

2- 400g cans diced tomatoes or 3 cups fresh tomatoes
2 tablespoons of olive oil
500g of lamb, diced
1 large onion, sliced thinly.
3 finely chopped garlic cloves
½ teaspoon caraway seeds
¼ cup of ground paprika

Instructions

With the oil in the pan add in the veal, set to medium heat and fry until browned. Save the pan juices to use as a sauce.

Remove veal from pan and add remaining oil along with garlic and onion. Put it on medium heating and cook veal for at least 4-5 minutes or until onions are soft. Add in the caraway seeds and paprika and stir for about 30 seconds.

Add in the veal and diced tomatoes to the pan, cover and leave to simmer for about an hour or until meat is tender and the sauce has thickened. If the sauce begins to dry then add in a little water to the mixture.

Moroccan Lamb with Squash

Ingredients

500g of lamb diced
1 tablespoon oil
Chicken or vegetable stock – 3 cups
1 tbsp ground cinnamon
3 cups of pumpkin diced
1 sliced onion
Cut into halves 6 yellow button squash
1 juiced lemon
1 tablespoon of honey
2/3 cups of prunes, pitted
Salt and pepper to taste

Instructions

In a pan heat oil, fry up the diced lamb until it has been cooked thoroughly.
Add in the chicken or vegetable stock and cinnamon. Cover the pan and simmer for at least an hour.

Add in the squash, onion, pumpkin, honey and lemon juice, then cover again and simmer for at least a half hour, or until vegetables have been cooked. Add in salt, pepper, and prunes, and cook for about 5 minutes.

Allow it to cook before serving.

Poultry

Chicken with Macadamia Topping

Ingredients

2 teaspoons of olive oil
2 chicken breasts cut into 3 parts

For the Macadamia Topping:

1/3 cup of red onion diced
1 chopped finely garlic clove
1 teaspoon of the oil of your choice
Salt
½ cup of macadamia nuts
4 tablespoons of chives, chopped

Instructions

Put the pan on high setting, fry chicken with the oil. Cook the chicken for about 5-11 minutes or until the chicken is cooked thoroughly and browned. Cook both sides of the chicken.

For the macadamia topping, fry the onion, salt, garlic and oil separately until the nuts are soft and browned. Remove ingredients from the pan but leave the oil in it. Put the pan back on the heat and add in the macadamia nuts. Stir the nuts regularly until they are browned lightly. Use a blender to mix garlic and onion and nuts and pulse the blender until a crunchy texture has developed. Put the mixture into a bowl and combine in the chopped chives.

Sprinkle a sizeable amount of the macadamia combination over the chicken on a plate.

Serve the dish with steamed vegetables and a green salad.

Orange Chicken with Basil

2 tablespoons of olive oil
1 cup of orange juice, freshly squeezed (used oranges)
2 chicken breasts
Sea salt
Fresh basil 2/3 cup chopped roughly

Instructions

Pre-heat oven to 350° degrees Fahrenheit.

Using 2 pieces of baking paper place the chicken breasts into them. Bash the chicken breasts with a meat hammer until they are at least 1cm thick. Use a meat hammer or the end of a rolling pin and bash chicken breasts until 1cm thick.

Place the chicken breasts into an oven dish along and add in the basil, olive oil, orange juice, and a good dash of sea salt. Using aluminum foil, cover the oven dish tightly. Bake in oven for about 30-40 minutes, or until it is cooked thoroughly.

Serve with a salad or steamed vegetables.

Avocado Sauce with Baked Chicken

Ingredients:

Largely chopped pumpkin at least 3 cups
1 tablespoon of olive oil
2 chicken breast fillets
½ of an avocado
1 tablespoon of finely chopped fresh basil
Salt and pepper
1 cup of fresh rocket leaves
1 tablespoon of lemon juice

Instructions:

Pre-heat oven to $350°$ degrees Fahrenheit.

In an dish oven proof, put the pumpkin, salt and pepper, and olive oil. Bake for approximately 35-60 minutes or until completely cooked.

In medium heat, put the olive oil in a pan, fry chicken for about 4-8 minutes on each side or until cooked completely. Set the chicken aside for 5 minutes, then cutting across the grain, slice the chicken thinly.

In a blender or food processor, put the basil, lemon juice

and avocado, pulse until a smooth paste has formed.

Put the chicken over the pumpkin and add the rocket leaves and add the avocado sauce.

Bombay Chicken Skewers

Ingredients

6 wooden skewers (soaked in cold water for about 20-30 minutes)
2 diced chicken breasts
4 tablespoons oil
2 tablespoons sweet paprika
1 tablespoon ground cumin
1 tablespoon ground coriander
2 finely chopped cloves of garlic
1 tablespoon ground turmeric

Instructions

Pre-heat oven to 350°degrees Fahrenheit or pre-heat grill on high setting.
To make sauce heat oil and spices in a frying pan on medium heat for 2-3 minutes, or until fragrant.

Line an oven tray with baking paper and then thread chicken on skewers. Coat chicken well with sauce.

Bake in oven for approximately 30-40 minutes, or until chicken has completely cooked.

Cook chicken for 4-7 minutes on each side if using a grill.

Rosemary and Lemon Chicken Skewers

Ingredients:

6 wooden skewers (soaked in cold water for about 20-30 minutes)
2 diced chicken breasts
2 tablespoons rosemary, finely chopped
2 tablespoons olive oil
1 tsp grated lemon rind
1/3 cup of lemon juice
Salt for taste

Instructions

Pre-heat oven to 350°degrees Fahrenheit or pre-heat BBQ grill on high.
Place rosemary, lemon rind, olive oil, lemon juice and salt in a small bowl and combine together.

Thread chicken on skewers and put in a tray oven proof lined with baking paper, coat the chicken with lemon sauce and rosemary. Bake in the oven for about 30-40 minutes, or until chicken has thoroughly cooked.

Cook chicken for 4-6 minutes on each side if cooking on a grill.

Snacks

Pistachio Salsa

Ingredients:

1/3 cup of toasted pistachios
1 cup finely diced tomatoes
1 finely chopped large garlic clove
1/3 cup of roughly chopped fresh parsley
2 finely chopped mint leaves,
1 tbsp of lemon juice
Dash of round paprika

Instructions:

Combine all ingredients in a bowl and mix together well.

Tomato Salsa

Ingredients:

1 cup finely diced tomato
¼ cup of finely chopped red onion
1 ½ tbsp of ground paprika
½ tsp of Mexican chili powder
1 tsp of finely chopped tarragon or oregano
1 tbsp lemon juice
1 tsp vinegar (optional)

Instructions:

Combine all ingredients in a bowl and mix together well.

Cashew Nut Dip

Ingredients:

2/3 cup of unsalted cashews
1 tbsp of olive oil
3 tbsp lemon juice
Salt and pepper for flavor

Instructions:

Use a blender to combine all of the ingredients together until a smooth paste has formed.

For a crunchy texture then blend the ingredients for a shorter period of time.

Desserts

Blueberry Sorbet
Ingredients
2 cups blueberries
½ medium banana
1/3 cup of coconut milk
1½ tbsp honey
1 egg white, beaten until stiff peaks have formed

Instructions

Use a blender to blend together blueberries, banana, coconut milk and honey until well combined.

Fold blueberry mixture into the beaten egg white. Pour into an ice-cream container or a freezer proof container and freeze for approximately 6 hours or overnight until set.

To serve, cut into slices.

Stir in shredded coconut and then fold mixture into the beaten egg white.

Pour the mixture into an ice-cream container / freezer

proof container and freeze for approximately 6 hours or overnight until set.

To serve, cut into slices and enjoy.

Mixed Berry Compote

Ingredients

2 tea bags herbal tea, such as chamomile, orange tea, jasmine
1 freshly squeezed orange
2 cups mixed berries

Instructions

Place tea bags and orange juice in a saucepan and simmer over low heat for 1 minute.

Add in the berries and allow it to simmer until berries are juicy and plump.

Take out the tea bags.

Cover and refrigerate for several hours prior to serving.

Paleolithic Cookbook Conclusion

The Paleo diet isn't a diet that is going to fade away but instead will continue to grow as more people gain knowledge about the full benefits of the diet. The fundamentals of the paleo diet provide dieters with the needed guidelines and principles to apply to our daily life and lifestyle. Our ancestors' diet may have varied as it depended on where they lived along with their environmental climates and other factors involved. Ancestors living around Canada would more likely eat fresh salmon, deer, berries and plants. Ancestors living in Africa would eat animals and plant roots. Aboriginals in Australia would live off the land eating plants, bugs, native nuts, honey and animals. Remember our ancestors ate well and were in good health and this same diet will provide the exact same benefits for us.

Lightning Source UK Ltd.
Milton Keynes UK
UKHW022100300920
370813UK00006B/670